Foreword:

Let me start by saying I'm not a doctor and
medical advice or treatment of any illness. T... ___..
hours of research and organization, not only to help myself, but to help my
friends and family in their quest for better health.

My cousin Joe Ann Murphy got me started in juicing, and pushed me to publish
this book (Thank you!). There is so much information out there on how to start
that it can be overwhelming. What I've tried to create is a condensed, clear and
concise book to get you started. There are tons of recipes for juices out there in
books and on the internet, but if you're just getting started, it just makes it all
that much more confusing! Even if you buy 100% natural, not from concentrate,
orange juice, if you do a little research you'll find out that the process they use
to preserve the juice takes out the flavor and color so they add artificial flavors
and colors right back in and call it natural! See page 66 for more details.

Use common sense. Consult your doctor to see if you're healthy enough to start
juicing. Have your doctor run some standard blood work on you, this can be your
"before" so you can tell everyone that your cholesterol is lower, blood pressure is
down, blood sugar levels are down, etc. Not only will the tests see if you're
healthy enough to start juicing, but it will give you a reference point to see your
progress! Take before photos too! Nothing is more motivational that to see
actual, physical results, of your hard work.
Above all, have fun and be creative!

Happy juicing!

Tina Swindell

Juicing for Beginners

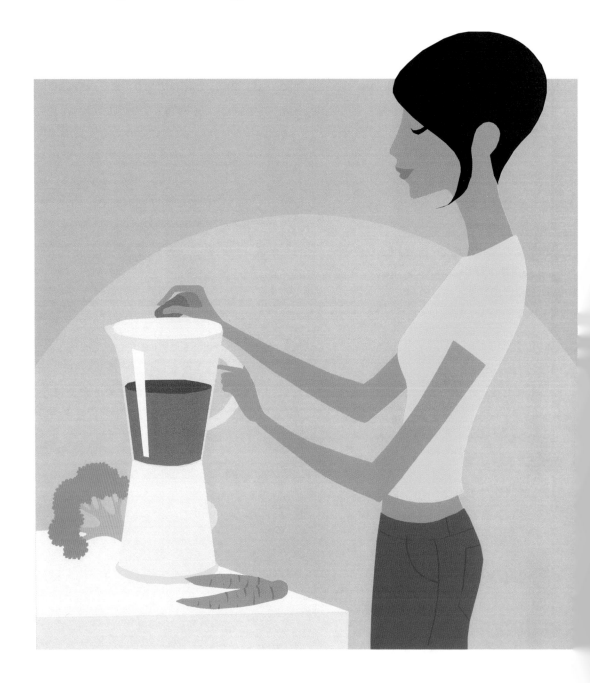

Table of Contents

Starting With a Clean Slate...

INTERNAL SALT WATER BATHING

Colon Cleanse – This helps cleanse the entire digestive tract and is inexpensive.

DIRECTIONS:

1 quart of lukewarm water
2 teaspoons of Pink Himalayan or Celtic Sea salt (not iodized)

Drink the entire quart of salt and water first thing in the morning on an empty stomach. Do this when you will be at home preferably, as you will likely eliminate several times. If it doesn't work the first time, try adding a little more or less salt until you find a balance that works for you. Increasing your intake of water will often increase the activity.

It is quite advisable to take the herb laxative tea at night to loosen, then the salt water each morning to help flush it out.

*Do not take supplements during the internal cleanse

Body Cleanse

- 2 apples (cored)
- 1 stalk of celery
- 1 slice of lemon with rind
- 1" piece of cucumber
- 1" slice of ginger root

Wash the fruits and vegetables thoroughly. Core and slice the apples. Remove the ends from the celery. Put all ingredients in a juicer. Serve over ice, if desired.

Coffee Enema for Liver Detoxification

A coffee enema is a simple, yet effective, way to cleanse our body. The liver is our primary processor of all the blood in the body. Coffee enema cleanses the toxins and wastes in the blood by stimulating the liver to make more bile.

Preparing the coffee:

o Mix 2 teaspoons of ground coffee and 2 cups of water in a pot; boil it for 10 minutes.

o Combine coffee mixture with 4 cups of purified or filtered water (6 cups total).

o Check mixture temperature to make sure it is no higher than 104° F. Use a thermometer or place your washed hand in it for 5 seconds to feel if it's too hot. This is important as you don't want to damage your internal organs.

Enema Instructions:

o Prepare your bathroom space to do the enema. Place a folded blanket or towel on the floor or even in the bathtub, near the toilet preferably. Play some relaxing music if you'd like. (Make sure there is something nearby to hang the enema bag from – door knob, shower door, cabinet, etc.)

o Pour mixture into a reusable enema bag or fill up a disposable enema bottle. If using a disposable bottle you will have to refill it several times during the process.

o Hang the bag on a door knob or something that is almost the same height (must be higher than your body for it to flow).

o Open the clamp and release some coffee out to make sure no air is in the tube.

o Put some olive oil, grapefruit oil, any oil that is not highly processed or a commercial personal lubricant on the end of the tube. Relax and slowly insert the tube 2 inches into your anus.

o Lie down on the floor on your left side, release the clamp and allow the coffee to start going in your body. Stay in this position for 10 to 15 minutes, holding the enema in.

o Finally, release the coffee into the toilet bowl. Several eliminations will likely occur so staying close to a bathroom is highly advisable

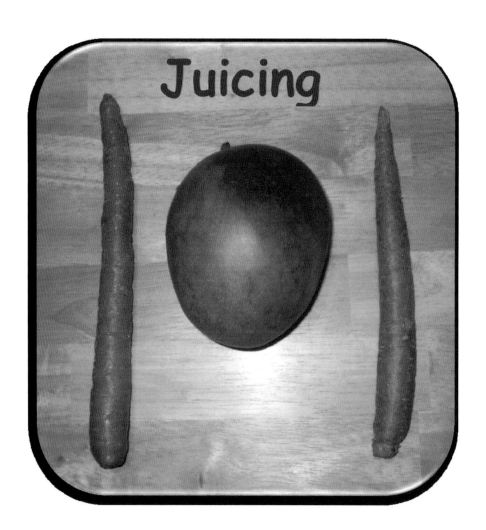

Why Juice?

- All green plants contain chlorophyll which stimulates blood production and nourishment, and promotes blood oxygenation which helps the body to cleanse itself. It also binds and releases toxins from where they were lodged inside the body so that they can be carried away and processed. Fruit and vegetable juice is an excellent source of vitamins & minerals, trace elements, enzymes and nutrients, all of which supply essential elements required for the body's healing processes and cell regeneration.
- Vegetable juices are rich in natural medicines, hormones and antibiotics.
- Fresh fruit and vegetable juice contains easily absorbed organic minerals such as calcium, potassium and silicon. These assist the body in restoring the chemical & mineral balance in the tissues & cells, which helps to prevent the premature aging of cells and disease.
- Raw, fresh vegetable juices are extremely alkaline. High acidity is the common theme and cause of almost all illness. Maintaining an alkaline balance in the blood and tissues helps ensure that your body does not become over-acidic.
- Cooking and processing food destroys micronutrients by altering their shape and chemical composition. Eating or drinking raw vegetables and fruit maintains the nutrients.

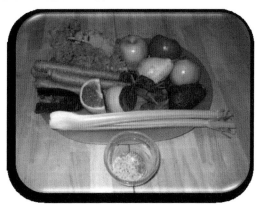

Imagine eating the above platter of food for dinner, uncooked (platter is 11-1/2" X 15-1/2"). The majority of plant matter is composed of cellulose which our bodies can't break down. With juicing you can pack all of that nutrition into a few cups of liquid, with no preservatives, artificial flavors, or sweeteners! Juicing allows you to extract all of the nutrition without the added bulk. By the way, that's the ingredients in the Lean & Green Juice on page 40!

Adding Juicing to Your Diet

As with any lifestyle change, you need to be sensible. This means that if you are doing a fast or cleanse, you need to take in enough calories for your body to function properly, and that you shouldn't feel hungry constantly. If you're actually juice fasting (cleansing), it takes at least two days for your body to clear all of your solid food from your body, so you need to juice for at least that long. Consult your doctor prior to starting a juice fast or any diet.

Here are some suggestions to make things a bit easier:

1. Juicing removes bulk (fiber) from your diet so be sure to add fiber back in with a supplement. If you have a high-speed blender such as a Vitamix® then it's not necessary to add fiber because you're drinking the pulp as well.
2. Use fresh, organic foods when possible. **<u>Always</u> wash your produce thoroughly** and refrigerate any unused portion in an airtight container. Ideally, drink juice immediately because the phytonutrients, enzymes and antioxidants start to break down quickly after they are extracted from the pulp. Expect to get about 8 ounces of juice per pound of produce.
3. Drinking a glass of water before you drink your juice can give you the extra water your body needs so your kidneys can flush all of the toxins and waste from your body. **Drink at least a gallon of water per day.** You shouldn't feel hungry or thirsty while juicing after the first few days. If you do, add a juice "snack" to your day. (I recommend the Apple Pie Juice recipe on pg. 32)
4. **If you're fasting, adding herbal teas is fine,** just don't add anything that has added caffeine, sugar, sodium or artificial sweeteners.
5. Before going on a juice fast, slowly **eliminate caffeine, dairy products and meat from your diet.** You don't want to traumatize your body by going from burger combo meals one day to organic veggies the next!
6. **Clean your juicer thoroughly every time that you use it.** Fresh fruits and vegetables are particularly attractive to bacteria that can make you sick! The pulp can be used in a compost bin so you can grow your own fruits and vegetables!
7. **Not all fruits are the same.** Not all juicers will work well with citrus fruits so you may want to purchase a separate citrus juicer for those. If your juice tastes bitter try peeling your citrus before juicing, as the pith (the white part between skin and pulp) has a bitter flavor. Also, apple seeds contain cyanide. Eaten whole, the seeds coating protects your body from the cyanide, but if you're juicing a lot of apples, you might consider seeding them first. An apple corer works wonders for this. Also, melon tends not to mix well with other fruit juices. Other fruits can easily be juiced together in any combination you like!

8. **Use fruits sparingly.** Adding fruit for sweetness is fine, but try to use mostly veggies as they're much lower in sugar and higher in nutrients. Since you're not getting any fiber to slow down the conversion of sugar to glycogen, you may experience spikes in your insulin levels which may cause your energy levels to crash.

9. **Sweeteners:** Not all fruits will work well with a heavy vegetable juice. If you are juicing with a nice blend of veggies try adding an apple to sweeten and save your other fruits for a nice fruity blend. You can also add agave nectar or honey for additional sweetness.

10. **Keep it simple.** Just pick 2-3 vegetables and perhaps toss in fruit or two for sweetness, and you will have delicious and nutritious juice. It's the same with fruits, picking just a couple to combine together will allow you to taste each fruit and enjoy the flavors. Think of it as cooking, you wouldn't throw 10 random items into a meal just because you have it on hand. **Drinking your juice prior to a meal is best.** Your body will absorb more of the nutrients and enzymes since the juice is sitting on an empty stomach and you will feel more full when you sit down to eat, which will help you control your portions so you eat less.

11. **Buy what's in season!** Make it a point every time you go to the grocery store to explore new options in the fresh produce department. Scour local farmers markets stop at those roadside stands where farmers direct sell their goods.

12. **Don't juice up the same thing every day.** Your body needs a wide variety of nutrients, so try different recipes. You can purchase in bulk for a week to save money, but make sure to change an ingredient or two every week. This will also keep you from getting bored with your juices.

13. **Some fruits and vegetables are not meant for juicing.** Soft fruits like bananas and avocados are best blended not juiced. Blend up a banana and add it to a fruit smoothie for a thicker, creamier consistency. You can always make fresh juice and then pour some into a blender with these fruits and vegetables for a nice smoothie.

14. **Leafy greens will work best if you squish them together prior to juicing.** Balling up leafy greens will help the juicer work best.

15. **Coffee filters** can be used to eliminate pulp if you don't like the texture in your juice.

16. **Colors!** Lemon juice eliminates color changes in fresh juice. Adding beetroot to your juice can cause your urine to turn pink and it's strong so start with half of a beetroot. Eating or drinking a lot of carrots can cause your skin to turn orange; although this isn't dangerous, most of us avoid looking like a giant carrot!

Ok, so you've read all of the good benefits of juicing and it sounds great, but there are some things you need to know before jumping right into juicing! You may experience some unpleasant side effects of juicing during the first few days, especially if you're replacing more than one meal with juice, because your body is ridding itself of accumulated wastes and toxins. Don't worry, this is temporary! Here are a few things you might experience when you start juicing:

- **A drop in energy for the first day or two may be expected** because the sugar levels in your blood will be lower since you're not consuming all of the carbs that your body is probably used to. Also, since you're drinking pure juice, the sugars that you are getting are rapidly absorbed which may cause your energy levels to fluctuate. If you're diabetic, you must pay special attention to what's going in your juice.
- **You may experience headaches,** especially if you're used to consuming caffeine and sugar on a regular basis. Just remember – a headache isn't caused by the orange-carrot juice that you had for breakfast. It's caused by the fact that your body is craving the bad stuff that it's used to!
- **Nausea or vomiting may occur** because your body isn't used to such high doses of nutrients without the accompanying fiber and protein. This may also be another withdrawal side effect or it may be a reaction to herbs or spices that you add. It can also be caused by the sheer concentration of some of the juices. If this happens, dilute your juice with pure water.
- **Bad breath, acne and/or body odor may occur** because your body is flushing out waste and toxins and two of the ways that your body does this is through your skin and through the exhalation process. These side effects should disappear within a few days. (Try the recipe for bad breath found on page 19)
- **You may experience constipation or diarrhea.** The constipation may be caused by the sudden lack of fiber so add a natural herbal laxative to your regimen while you're juicing and drink lots of water. Diarrhea may occur because you're not eating as much solid foods and your digestive tract is being cleansed. If you experience more than temporary diarrhea for a day, you may want to add some fiber back into your diet because you can become dehydrated.

If any of these side effects linger for more than the first few days, or if they are severe, stop juicing and talk to your doctor immediately.

Don't Give Up!

Fruit & Vegetable Storage 101

Great tasting fruits and vegetables begin with proper storage at home. Rotate your stock to where the oldest is eaten first to ensure freshness and reduce waste. This applies to all types of foods—fresh, frozen, canned and dried. If you have a vacuum-type food storage system, please consult your owner's manual for storage times, otherwise the charts below are a good guideline.

Fruit	Room Temp. (70° F)	Refrigerator (37°-40° F)	Freezer (0 ° F)	Additional Info
Apples		3-5 months	4-6 months	Core & slice
Apricots		3-5 days	6 months	
Avocados	2-3 days if ripe	5-10 days		
Bananas	Varies by ripeness		6 months	Freeze whole in skin or peel and mash
Berries		2-3 days	6 months	Freeze individually on cookie sheets then place in plastic bags
Cherries		2-3 days	6 months	Freeze individually on cookie sheets then place in plastic bags
Cranberries		3-4 weeks	4-6 months	
Grapefruit	7 days	2 weeks	4-6 months	Wrap cut surface
Grapes		1-2 weeks	4-6 months	Freeze individually on cookie sheets then place in plastic bags
Guavas		1-2 days		
Kiwi	3-5 days after ripe	4-6 months if not ripe		
Lemons	1 week	2-5 weeks	4-6 months	Quarter and freeze individually on cookie sheets then place in plastic bags
Limes	1 week	2-5 weeks	4-6 months	*same as lemons
Melons		1 week	8-12 months	Wrap cut surfaces to prevent Vitamin C loss
Papayas		1-2 days		
Nectarines		3-5 days	6 months	
Oranges	3-4 days	5-6 weeks		
Peaches	room temp.	2-3 days	6 months	
Pears		3-5 days	6 months	
Pineapple	1-2 days	3-5 days	6 months	
Plums		3-5 days	6 months	
Tangerines	2-3 days	1 week		
Watermelon	Uncut 2-3 days	6-8 days	8-12 months	

Vegetable	Room Temp. (70° F)	Refrigerator (37°-40° F)	Freezer (0 ° F)	Additional Info
Artichokes		1 week		
Asparagus		3-5 days	8-12 months	
Beans		3-6 days	8-12 months	
Beets		2 weeks	8-12 months	
Broccoli		3-6 days	8-12 months	
Bell peppers		1-2 weeks	3-4 months	Freeze raw
Cabbage		1 week	Do not freeze	
Carrots		2 weeks	8-12 months	
Cauliflower		1 week	8-12 months	
Celery		1 week	8-12 months	
Chilies		1 week	8-12 months	
Collard Greens		3-5 days	8-12 months	
Corn		immediately	8-12 months	
Cucumber		3-5 days		
Green Onions		3-5 days	Do not freeze	Becomes limp if frozen
Green Beans		3-5 days	8-12 months	
Kale		3-5 days	8-12 months	
Lettuce		1 week	Do not freeze	Too watery to freeze
Mushrooms		1-2 days	8-12 months	Slice & sauté first
Mustard		3-5 days	8-12 months	
Radishes		2 weeks		
Spinach		3-5 days	8-12 months	
Squash	3-6 months			
Swiss Chard		3-5 days	8-12 months	
Tomatoes	depends on ripeness		3-4 months	Cut in wedges

Homemade Fruit & Vegetable Wash/Soak

SPRAY Ingredients:
- 1 tablespoon fresh lemon juice
- 1 tablespoon baking soda

Directions:
Put all ingredients into a spray bottle; shake gently to mix. Spray on veggies or fruit; wait 2-5 minutes then rinse under cold water.

SOAK Ingredients
- 1/4 cup vinegar
- 2 tablespoons salt
- 1 cup water

Directions:
Add ingredients in large bowl or sink. Soak fruit and/or veggies for 25-30 minutes. Rinse under cold water and dry.

What's in Season?

Spring	Summer		Winter
Apricots	Apples	Figs	Beets
Artichokes	Apricots	Garlic	Broccoli
Arugula	Avocados	Grapes	Brussels
Asparagus	Basil	Green beans	sprouts
Beets	Beets	Horseradish	Cabbage
Carrots	Blackberries	Kale	Cardoons
Chard	Blueberries	Kohlrabi	Carrots
Cherries	Boysenberries	Leeks	Cauliflower
Fava beans	Cantaloupes	Lemongrass	Celery root
Fennel	Carrots	Lettuce	Clementine
Fiddleheads	Chard	Limes	Escarole
Garlic	Cherries	Mushrooms	Fennel
Grapefruit	Chiles, fresh	Okra	Grapefruit
Green onions	Corn	Onions	Horseradish
Greens	Cucumbers	Parsnips	Artichokes
Kohlrabi	**Autumn**	Pears	Kale
Kumquats	Apples	Peppers	Kiwi
Leeks	Artichokes	Persimmons	Kohlrabi
Lemons	Arugula	Pomegranates	Kumquats
Lettuce	Beets	Potatoes	Leeks
Morels	Broccoli	Pumpkins	Lemons
Nettles	Broccoli raabe,	Quinces	Mandarins
Spring onions	rapini	Radicchio	Onions
Navel oranges	Brussels	Radishes	Oranges
Parsley	sprouts	Rapini	Parsnips
Pea greens	Cabbage	Rutabaga	Pommels
Peas	Carrots	Salsify	Potatoes
Radishes	Cauliflower	Scallions	Radishes
Rhubarb	Celeriac/Celery	Shallots	Rutabaga
Spinach	Chard	Shelling beans	Salsify
Strawberries	Cranberries	Sweet potatoes	Shallots
Turnips	Edamame	Turnips	Sweet Potatoes
	Eggplant	Winter squash	Tangerines
	Fennel		Winter squash

Buy Organic!

You get up every morning and make your delicious healthy juice, making sure to use only fresh ingredients, even buying what's in season to save money. Sounds healthy right? But did you add pesticides and other toxic chemicals as well? Unless you buy only organic, you probably did! Don't sabotage your efforts by adding harmful chemicals to your juice. If you can't afford to buy all organic produce at least try to buy these organically grown since they are the worst for containing pesticides.

Apples	Grapes
Celery	Sweet Bell Peppers
Strawberries	Blueberries
Peaches	Lettuce
Spinach	Kale/Collard Greens
Cilantro	Sweet Potatoes
Potatoes	Oranges
Nectarines (imported)	Cucumbers

Source: USDA Pesticide Data Program, Annual Summary, Calendar year 2009
Pages 181-183

Education is the key to good health. Read up on how things are grown and processed. Organic means that no pesticides or chemicals were used in the growing process, however, it does not cover packaging and shipping. Pay attention to labels. There are several great documentaries out there and here are a few I highly recommend (they are available on Netflix on demand/DVD and Youtube.com for viewing or for purchase)

Fat, Sick, and Nearly Dead (A great inspiration for juicing!)
Food Matters
Food, Inc.

These are just a few! It'll change the way you look at food! Take charge of your health and feel better!

Ailments

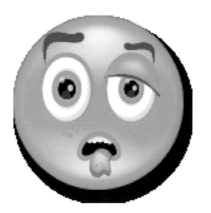

Acidity

Fruits & Veggies to add to your diet:

- ✓ Beetroot
- ✓ Carrot
- ✓ Celery
- ✓ Grape
- ✓ Lettuce

- ✓ Orange
- ✓ Peach
- ✓ Pear
- ✓ Spinach
- ✓ Tomato

Recipe:

- 3 carrots
- 2 stalks celery
- 4-6 leaves of lettuce or winter greens
- A handful of spinach or watercress (or dandelion) leaves
- A few stalks of fresh coriander or parsley

✺ -- ✺

Acne

Fruits & Veggies to add to your diet:

- ✓ Apricot
- ✓ Broccoli
- ✓ Carrot
- ✓ Celery
- ✓ Grapefruit

- ✓ Mango
- ✓ Melon
- ✓ Onion
- ✓ Orange
- ✓ Pumpkin

- ✓ Spinach
- ✓ Strawberry
- ✓ Watercress

Recipe 1:
- 3 carrots
- 1 apple (cored)

Recipe 2:
- 1 cup of broccoli heads
- 1/2 apple (cored)
- 3 carrots

Recipe 3:
- 1 cup of blueberries
- 1 cup of blackberries
- 3 kiwis (peeled)

> ➤ These are high in Vitamin A, E and Zinc which can be helpful in preventing inflammation and flare ups in the skin. Zinc is also an important mineral needed for skin to heal and to reduce the effects of scarring.

Age (anti-aging foods)

Fruits & Veggies to add to your diet:

- ✓ Apple
- ✓ Apricot
- ✓ Avocado
- ✓ Blackberry
- ✓ Blueberry
- ✓ Broccoli
- ✓ Cabbage
- ✓ Cranberry
- ✓ Garlic
- ✓ Gooseberry
- ✓ Grape
- ✓ Kale
- ✓ Lettuce
- ✓ Radish
- ✓ Spinach
- ✓ Tomato

Recipe 1:
- 4 carrots
- 3 stalks celery
- 1 handful of spinach
- 1 small piece of onion
- 1/4" ginger root (peeled)

Recipe 2:
- 4 carrots
- 1/2 cup of broccoli
- 1 handful of spinach
- 1/2 cucumber
- 1 clove garlic

Recipe 3:
- 1 apple (cored)
- 1/5 cabbage
- 1 handful of spinach
- 1/4" ginger root (peeled)

Recipe 4:
- 2 tomatoes
- 5 stalks celery
- 1 bunch parsley
- 1 squeeze of lemon

Recipe 5:
- 4 carrots
- 1 handful of string beans
- 1/2 cucumber

Recipe 6:
- 1 cucumber
- 5 stalks celery
- 1/4 beet

Recipe 7:
- 5 carrots
- 4 kale leaves
- 1 handful of parsley
- 1/2 apple (cored)

Allergies

Fruits & Veggies to add to your diet:
- ✓ Carrot
- ✓ Pineapple

Recipe 1:
- 3 carrot2
- 2 celery stalks
- 1/4 cup pineapple (cored & peeled)
- 1/2 beetroot

Recipe 2:
- 4 cups of pineapple (cored & peeled)
- 1/2 beetroot

Recipe 3:
- 1 - 2 cups of pineapple (cored & peeled)
- 2 large carrots

➢ Pineapple contains bromelain (enzyme), which is used as a treatment for inflammation and swelling of the nose, ear, and sinuses.

Alzheimer's

Fruits & Veggies to add to your diet:
- ✓ Alfalfa Sprouts
- ✓ Beets
- ✓ Blackberries
- ✓ Blueberries
- ✓ Broccoli
- ✓ Cabbage
- ✓ Carrot
- ✓ Cherries
- ✓ Grapes (Red)
- ✓ Kale
- ✓ Kelp
- ✓ Lettuce
- ✓ Onion
- ✓ Oranges
- ✓ Pumpkin
- ✓ Raspberries
- ✓ Spinach
- ✓ Strawberries
- ✓ Watercress

Recipe 1:
- 2 cups of strawberries
- 2 cups of blueberries
- 1-1/2 cups of raspberries

Recipe 2:
- 1 cup of spinach
- 1/2 cucumber
- 2 stalks of celery (including leaves)
- 3 carrots
- 1/2 apple (cored)

➢ Current research suggests that certain foods, such as dark-skinned fruits and vegetables may reduce the risk of heart disease and stroke, and appear to protect brain cells.

✂ -- ✂

Anemia

Fruits & Veggies to add to your diet:

- ✓ Apricot
- ✓ Beetroot
- ✓ Carrot
- ✓ Cherry
- ✓ Dandelion Leaves
- ✓ Figs
- ✓ Grapefruit
- ✓ Grapes
- ✓ Kiwi Fruit
- ✓ Lemon
- ✓ Lettuce
- ✓ Lime
- ✓ Oranges
- ✓ Parsley
- ✓ Prune
- ✓ Raisins
- ✓ Spinach
- ✓ Strawberry
- ✓ Turnip Leaves
- ✓ Watercress

Recipe:

- • 6 carrots
- • 1/2 beetroot
- • 1/4 cup celery
- • 1/4 cup lettuce
- • 1 apple (cored)

➢ In Europe, beet juice has been used as a treatment for anemia. It contains iron, folic acid, Vitamin B1, B2, B6, and vitamins A & C.

✂ -- ✂

Anxiety

Fruits & Veggies to add to your diet:

- ✓ Broccoli
- ✓ Celery
- ✓ Lemon
- ✓ Lettuce
- ✓ Lime
- ✓ Orange
- ✓ Peach
- ✓ Spinach
- ✓ Tomato
- ✓ Watercress

Recipe:

- • 4 small Granny Smith apples (cored)
- • 3 medium sized carrots
- • 4 stalks of celery

➢ B Vitamins have been shown to have a wide range of benefits in mood, memory, mental clarity and energy.

∽ --- ✺

Arthritis

Fruits & Veggies to add to your diet:

- ✓ Apple
- ✓ Broccoli
- ✓ Carrot
- ✓ Celery

- ✓ Cucumber
- ✓ Grape
- ✓ Lemon
- ✓ Pear

- ✓ Pineapple
- ✓ Red Pepper
- ✓ Tomato

Recipe:

- 6 carrots
- 3 stalks of celery
- 1/4 cup pineapple (peeled & cored)
- 1 oz. lemon

➢ Fresh pineapple contains bromelain (enzyme) which works as a natural anti-inflammatory substance for swollen and painful joints.

∽ --- ✺

Asthma

Fruits & Veggies to add to your diet:

- ✓ Alfalfa Sprouts
- ✓ Apricot
- ✓ Carrot

- ✓ Celery
- ✓ Grapes
- ✓ Orange
- ✓ Parsley

- ✓ Pear
- ✓ Pepper (Red)
- ✓ Wheatgrass

Recipe 1:

- 1 cup blueberries
- 1 cup blackberries
- 1 cup strawberries
- 1 cup grapes
- 1 lemon
- 1" slice ginger
- 4 carrots

Recipe 2:

- 4 carrots
- 1 apple (cored)
- 1 stalk celery
- 1/2 lemon
- 4 kale leaves

Recipe 3:

- 1 bunch nettle
- 1 cup broccoli
- 4 carrots

➢ Grapes have very potent anti-inflammatory properties. A diet that is high in chlorophyll helps promote detoxification of the liver and colon and along with it reduce the sensitivity to inflammation. Carrot is one of the best foods in dispelling excessive mucus from the body. Hot, pungent foods that provide immediate relief include: chili peppers, spicy mustard, garlic and onions. These foods have anti-asthmatic and anti-inflammatory properties.

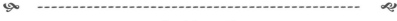

Bad breath

Fruits & Veggies to add to your diet:

- ✓ Apple
- ✓ Broccoli
- ✓ Carrot
- ✓ Fennel
- ✓ Parsley
- ✓ Pear
- ✓ Spinach
- ✓ Citrus Fruits

Recipe:

- • 6 carrots
- • 3-1/2 oz. (100 g) parsley

> ➢ Chewing parsley or mint leaves has been a remedy used for thousands of years. These herbs are especially good if garlic and onions are the source of your bad breath. Parsley is very high in chlorophyll.

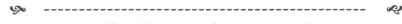

Blood Pressure (Hypertension)

Fruits & Veggies to add to your diet:

- ✓ Cabbage
- ✓ Celery
- ✓ Cucumber
- ✓ Dandelion
- ✓ Garlic
- ✓ Grapefruit
- ✓ Lemon
- ✓ Orange
- ✓ Parsley
- ✓ Pear

Recipe:

- • 8 carrots
- • 4 cloves of garlic

> ➢ Eating garlic lowers blood pressure and cholesterol levels, thereby reducing the risk of cardiovascular disease.

Blood cleansers

Fruits & Veggies to add to your diet:

✓ Beetroot	✓ Leafy Greens
✓ Carrot	✓ Lemon
✓ Dandelion	✓ Parsley
✓ Grapefruit	✓ Pineapple

Recipe:
- 3 carrots
- 3 stalks celery
- 1/4 small beet
- 1/2 tsp. lemon juice
- 1/4 tsp. ginger root (finely chopped)

Bronchitis

Fruits & Veggies to add to your diet:

✓ Carrot	✓ Onion
✓ Grape	✓ Orange
✓ Leek	✓ Spinach
✓ Lemon	

Recipe:
- 8 carrots
- 1/2 small de-seeded chili
- 2 cups fresh pineapple (cored & peeled)
- 1/2 lime
- 1 Tbsp. chopped coriander leaves

> ➢ Vitamin C, which is great for fighting off bronchial illness. Enzymes in the pineapple dissolve mucus, and the chili is a great expectorant. Chilies are rich in carotenoids and vitamin C, and are thought to help increase blood flow. They also have antibacterial properties which make them a favorite for beating colds and flu.

Cancer

Fruits & Veggies to add to your diet:

- ✓ Avocado
- ✓ Blackberry
- ✓ Blueberry
- ✓ Broccoli
- ✓ Brussels Sprouts
- ✓ Cabbage
- ✓ Carrot
- ✓ Cauliflower
- ✓ Chili Pepper
- ✓ Fig
- ✓ Garlic
- ✓ Grape (Red)
- ✓ Grapefruit
- ✓ Kale
- ✓ Leek
- ✓ Lemon
- ✓ Onion
- ✓ Orange
- ✓ Papaya
- ✓ Pumpkin
- ✓ Raspberry
- ✓ Spinach
- ✓ Strawberry
- ✓ Tomato
- ✓ Watercress

Recipe 1:
- 6 oz. pomegranate
- 2 oz. of water

Recipe 2:
- 4 carrots
- 1/2 cup cabbage
- 1/2 beetroot

➢ Pomegranate has more anti-oxidants than both green tea and red wine. Pomegranate juice can suppress the growth of prostate cancer cells due to ellagitannins – shown to have super anti-inflammatory powers. A 2005 study from the American Association for Cancer Research suggests that cabbage decreases cell mutation and DNA damage due to cabbage's anti-carcinogenic compound – glucosinolates.

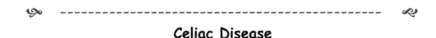

Celiac Disease

Fruits & Veggies to add to your diet:

- ✓ All fresh fruits and vegetables are naturally gluten-free so try different ones to see what works for you

Recipe:
- 4 carrots
- 1/4 cup kale
- 1 oz. fresh Aloe Vera (pulp not skin)

➢ A study shows that aloe promotes great gastrointestinal comfort and improves digestion/absorption.

Cholesterol

Fruits & Veggies to add to your diet:

- ✓ Apple
- ✓ Avocado
- ✓ Beans
- ✓ Blueberry
- ✓ Carrot
- ✓ Cranberry
- ✓ Garlic
- ✓ Kale
- ✓ Kiwi
- ✓ Onion
- ✓ Orange
- ✓ Swiss Chard
- ✓ Sweet Corn

Recipe 1:
- 2 apples (cored)
- 1 cucumber
- 1 stalk of celery

Recipe 2:
- 4 carrots
- 1 apple (cored)
- ¼" slice of ginger
- handful of parsley to taste
- Add a clove of garlic (optional)

Recipe 3:
- 2 celery stalks
- 1/2 bunch of spinach
- 2 carrots

* If you'd like the mixture to be a bit sweeter, add a splash of orange juice or 1/4 of an apple

Recipe 4:
- 1 medium-sized broccoli floret
- 1 small bunch of kale and
- 4 cups watermelon, cubed

➤ Juices made from apples and celery are known to fight cancer and reduce cholesterol. Spinach is full of anti-oxidants, which help keep cholesterol at healthy levels.

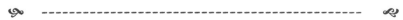

Cold, Fever and Flu

Recipe 1:
- 4 carrots
- 1 orange
- 1/4 lemon
- 4 cloves of garlic

Recipe 2:
- 1 cup pineapple (cored & peeled)
- 1/2 orange
- 4 fresh strawberries
- 1 bunch of red grapes

➤ Carrots, orange and lemon are great sources of natural form of vitamin C. Garlic is well known as nature's antibiotic and can prevent the common cold and aid in faster recovery.

Colitis, Crohn's Disease and Irritable Bowel Syndrome

Fruits & Veggies to add to your diet:

- ✓ Apricot
- ✓ Banana
- ✓ Cabbage
- ✓ Carrot
- ✓ Cherries
- ✓ Grapefruit
- ✓ Lettuce
- ✓ Orange
- ✓ Peach
- ✓ Pineapple
- ✓ Sweet Potato
- ✓ Tangerine
- ✓ Tomato
- ✓ Wheat Grass

Recipe1:
- 6 carrots
- 1/2 cup cabbage

Recipe 2:
- 6 carrots
- 2 oz. Wheat grass juice

➢ Wheat grass juice removes toxins and harmful bacteria from colon. Most peeled root vegetables contain soluble fiber. Not all juicers can juice wheat grass, check your owner's manual before trying.

Constipation

Fruits & Veggies to add to your diet:

- ✓ Apple
- ✓ Beetroot
- ✓ Blackberry
- ✓ Brussels Sprouts
- ✓ Carrot
- ✓ Cabbage
- ✓ Fennel
- ✓ Fig
- ✓ Grape
- ✓ Lettuce
- ✓ Orange
- ✓ Papaya
- ✓ Parsnip
- ✓ Peach
- ✓ Prune
- ✓ Pumpkin
- ✓ Sweet Corn

Recipe 1:
- 1 cup prunes
- 3 cups water

Soak overnight. Drink 8 oz. of the prune water on empty stomach.

Recipe 2:
- 1 pear
- 3 stalks of celery
- 1" piece of ginger root

➢ Prune juice promotes regular bowel movements, prevents constipation, and contains iron, which is great for people who are anemic or do not have enough iron in their system. Prunes are also much safer than over the counter laxatives.

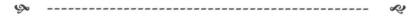

Cystic Fibrosis

Fruits & Veggies to add to your diet:
- ✓ Fruits & Veggies that contain Vitamins A, D, E and K and Calcium (See charts in Vitamins & Minerals Section)

Recipe:
- 5 carrots
- 1/2 cup of fresh cubed pineapple (cored & peeled)
- 1 lemon
- 5 cloves of garlic

> ➤ This juice effectively dissolves mucus, kills bacteria, and improves body's resistance to lung and sinus infections. Also, fresh pineapple is high in enzyme bromelain, which can literally digest not only protein but also old, sickly cells. This juice can help CS patients to thin and expel thick, nasty mucus thereby reducing the frequency of lung and sinus infections and constant need for antibiotics.

Cystitis

Fruits & Veggies to add to your diet:
- ✓ Blueberries
- ✓ Carrots
- ✓ Celery
- ✓ Coconuts
- ✓ Cranberries
- ✓ Cucumber
- ✓ Grapes
- ✓ Radish Sprouts
- ✓ Spinach

Recipe 1:
- 1/2 cup cranberries
- 2 celery sticks
- 1 apple
- 1 grapefruit
- 1 clove of garlic
- 3/4 cup cucumber
- 1 radish

Recipe 2:
- 1 lb. fresh cranberries
- 4 apples (cored)
- 2 pears

> ➤ Try adding garlic, cayenne, chia sprouts, flaxseed, coconut water/milk and alfalfa sprouts to your diet to help keep urinary tract infections at bay!

Diabetes

Fruits & Veggies to add to your diet:

- ✓ Asparagus
- ✓ Bitter Melon
- ✓ Broccoli
- ✓ Carrot
- ✓ Mangos
- ✓ Squash
- ✓ Tomatoes
- ✓ Sweet Potatoes
- ✓ Watermelon

Recipe:
- 3 oz. bitter melon
- 2 stalks celery
- 1/2 cup lettuce

> ➢ Broccoli is a non-starchy vegetable. It is one of the best choices for a diabetic because it is low in calories and antioxidant-rich with high amounts of vitamin C, vitamin A, beta-carotene and folic acid.

❧ --- ❧

Digestive disorders

Fruits & Veggies to add to your diet:

- ✓ Apple
- ✓ Beetroot
- ✓ Carrot
- ✓ Fennel
- ✓ Grape
- ✓ Kiwi
- ✓ Lemon
- ✓ Lettuce
- ✓ Orange
- ✓ Papaya
- ✓ Peach
- ✓ Pineapple
- ✓ Spinach

Recipe:
- 1 banana
- 1 apple (cored)
- Greens (kale, Swiss chard, spinach)
- 1 rounded Tbsp. chia seeds

Energy (Lack Of)

Fruits & Veggies to add to your diet:

- ✓ Apple
- ✓ Apricot
- ✓ Blueberry
- ✓ Cantaloupe Melon
- ✓ Carrot
- ✓ Fennel

- ✓ Grape
- ✓ Lemon
- ✓ Mango
- ✓ Parsley
- ✓ Parsnip
- ✓ Peach
- ✓ Pear

- ✓ Peppers
- ✓ Orange
- ✓ Spinach
- ✓ Strawberry
- ✓ Spinach

Recipe 1:
- · 2 apples (cored)
- · 1/2 cucumber
- · 1/2 lemon (peeled)
- · 1/2 cup of kale
- · 1/2 cup of spinach
- · 1/4 bunch of celery
- · 1/4 bulb of fennel
- · 1" slice of ginger
- · 1/4 head of romaine lettuce

Recipe 2:
- · 4 apples (cored)
- · 2 parsnips

➢ Lack of energy could be a sign of a serious illness. Consult your physician if this problem is persistent.

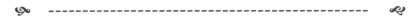

Hangover

Recipe:
- • 2 mangos (peeled with pit removed)
- • 1 pineapple (cored & peeled)

Heart Disease

Fruits & Veggies to add to your diet:

- ✓ Apple
- ✓ Beetroot
- ✓ Blackberry
- ✓ Broccoli *
- ✓ Carrot
- ✓ Cauliflower
- ✓ Celery
- ✓ Dandelion

- ✓ Garlic
- ✓ Green Pepper
- ✓ Grape
- ✓ Grapefruit
- ✓ Lettuce
- ✓ Melons
- ✓ Onion
- ✓ Orange

- ✓ Parsley *
- ✓ Pumpkin
- ✓ Spinach *
- ✓ Sweet Potato
- ✓ Tomato
- ✓ Watercress

Recipe:
- 1 cucumber
- 1 carrot
- 1 green apple (cored)
- 1/4 cup parsley
- 1/4 cup mint
- 1 stalk of celery
- 1/2" slice of fresh ginger
- 1/2 lemon (peeled)

➢ Vegetables marked with an asterisk * are high in Vitamin K and should be avoided if taking Coumadin.

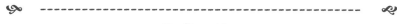

Indigestion

Fruits & Veggies to add to your diet:
- ✓ Papaya
- ✓ Pineapple

Recipe:
- 4 slices pineapple (peeled & cored)
- 2 apples (cored)
- 1 papaya (halve papaya, discard seeds and scoop out flesh)

➢ Papaya is great for acid reflux and indigestion

Kidney Stones

Recipe:
- 1/2 cup cranberry juice
- 1/2 cup water

Drink 3 times daily.

> ➢ Daily drinking of cranberry juice significantly decreases the formation of kidney stones (especially calcium oxalate).

࿊ --- ࿇

Prostate (enlarged or inflamed)

Recipe: Pomegranate 8oz

> ➢ Researchers from the Jonsson Cancer Center tested 50 men who had undergone treatment for prostate cancer, but whose cancer was still progressing. Drinking 8oz of pomegranate juice a day slowed the progression of cancer almost four-fold in 80% of the men. The researchers speculate that the results are a cause of the combination of antioxidants, polyphenols, and isoflavones found in pomegranate juice.

࿊ --- ࿇

Restless Leg Syndrome

Fruits & Veggies to add to your diet:

- ✓ Avocado
- ✓ Beetroot
- ✓ Bok Choy
- ✓ Blackberries
- ✓ Boysenberries
- ✓ Breadfruit
- ✓ Broccoli
- ✓ Chinese Cabbage
- ✓ Dates
- ✓ Guava
- ✓ Loganberries
- ✓ Mango
- ✓ Orange
- ✓ Papaya
- ✓ Passion fruit
- ✓ Peas
- ✓ Pineapple
- ✓ Pomegranate
- ✓ Potatoes
- ✓ Raspberries
- ✓ Spinach
- ✓ Squash – Summer & Winter
- ✓ Strawberries

Recipe:
- 2 cups strawberries
- 2 cups blueberries
- 1 orange
- 1 mango

> ➢ Studies have shown that sufferers of restless leg syndrome (RLS) have a deficiency in Folate (B9)

Rheumatism

Fruits & Veggies to add to your diet:

- ✓ Apple
- ✓ Cherry
- ✓ Lemon
- ✓ Pear
- ✓ Pineapple
- ✓ Tomato
- ✓ Carrot
- ✓ Celery
- ✓ Parsley
- ✓ Cucumber
- ✓ Tomato
- ✓ Watercress

Recipe 1:
- 3 kiwis (peeled)
- 3 cups of blackberries

Recipe 2:
- 4 carrots
- 1 apple (cored)

Recipe 3:
- 1/2 cucumber
- 2 carrots
- 1 cup of spinach
- 1 cup of kale
- 1/2 apple

Skin

Fruits & Veggies to add to your diet:

- ✓ Apricots
- ✓ Beets
- ✓ Bell Peppers
- ✓ Blackberries
- ✓ Blueberries
- ✓ Broccoli
- ✓ Cabbage
- ✓ Carrots
- ✓ Collards
- ✓ Cranberries
- ✓ Guava
- ✓ Kale
- ✓ Kiwi
- ✓ Mango
- ✓ Orange
- ✓ Papaya
- ✓ Pink Grapefruit
- ✓ Plums
- ✓ Purple Cabbage
- ✓ Red Grapes
- ✓ Red onions
- ✓ Romaine
- ✓ Strawberries
- ✓ Spinach
- ✓ Sweet Potatoes
- ✓ Tangerine
- ✓ Tomato
- ✓ Watermelon
- ✓ Winter Squash

Recipe 1:
- 3 apples (cored)
- 3 oranges

Recipe 2:
- 1/4 Watermelon (without rind)
- Sparkling Water to taste
- 1 Orange

Recipe 3:
- 1 cup of blueberries
- 1 cup of blackberries
- 1 cup of raspberries
- 1 cup of strawberries

➢ Vitamin C is great for the skin.

Upset Stomach

- 1 fennel bulb
- 8 Fl Oz. (240 Ml) water
- Small amount of fresh ginger or sprinkle of powdered ginger

Cut the fennel into slices and pass through the juicer. Add the water and a sprinkling of ginger.

∽ --- ✍

Weight Loss

Fruits & Veggies to add to your diet:

- ✓ Apples
- ✓ Beetroot
- ✓ Carrots
- ✓ Cherries
- ✓ Cucumbers
- ✓ Endive
- ✓ Escarole
- ✓ Grapefruits

- ✓ Kohlrabi
- ✓ Jerusalem Artichokes
- ✓ Lemons
- ✓ Lettuce (Bibb, Butter Crunch & Romaine)
- ✓ Pineapple

- ✓ Prunes
- ✓ Spinach
- ✓ Tomato
- ✓ Watercress

Recipe 1:
- 1 cup pineapple (peeled & cored)
- 1/2 cup broccoli
- 1/2 cup cucumber
- 1 kiwi

Recipe 2:
- 1 cup carrot
- 1 cup pineapple (peeled & cored)
- 1/2 lime (peeled)
- 1/2 small chili

Recipe 3:
- 2 oranges
- 1/2 lemon
- 1/2 cup beetroot
- 1/2 cup spinach
- 1/2 cup celery
- 1/2 cup carrot
- 1" slice of ginger root

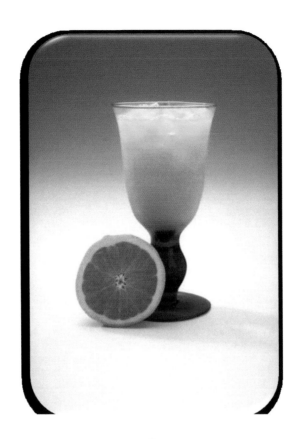

Juice

Recipes

These are just a few of the thousands of juice recipes to help get you started. Be creative and try new flavor combinations! Make most of your juices with veggies for maximum health benefits.

ABCs

- 2 Asian pears
- 2 apples (cored)
- 2 beets
- 2 carrots
- 1 cup cabbage (any variety)
- 6 handfuls Swiss chard (3 cups)

Apple-Carrot Juice

- 1 apple (cored)
- 2 carrots
- 1" slice of ginger
- 1 lemon

Apple-Cucumber Breakfast Juice

- 1 apple (cored)
- 1 cucumber
- 1" slice ginger
- 2 carrots

Apple-Carrot-Beet

- 2 apples (cored)
- 4 carrots
- 2 beets
- 6 leaves Swiss chard
- 1" slice ginger (1 tablespoon)

Apple- Lemon Juice

- 2 apples (cored)
- 1 wedge red cabbage
- 2 large carrots
- 1 piece ginger (thumb sized)
- 6 leaves Swiss chard
- 1/4 lemon

Apple Mix

- 2 apples (cored)
- 1/2 cantaloupe
- 1/2 honeydew
- 6 leaves kale
- 6 leaves Swiss chard

Apple Pie Juice

- $\frac{1}{2}$ tsp. of cinnamon
- $\frac{1}{2}$ tsp. of nutmeg
- 2 large sweet apples (cored)
- 2 green apples (cored)
- 3 carrots

Serve over ice and drink immediately. Makes 2 cups.

* This juice is good for eyes, skin, hair, ulcers, regularity, detoxification, colds and flu and tastes so good!

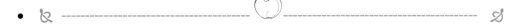

Beet, Celeriac, Carrot Juice

- 4 carrots
- 1 apple (cored)
- 1/2 celeriac root
- 1/2 beetroot
- 1/4" slice ginger root (optional)

Blackberry Kiwi

- 1/4 large pineapple (peeled & cored)
- 1 cup blackberries
- 1 kiwi fruit (peeled)
- 1/4 Comice pear
- 1/4 cup coconut water
- 30 mint leaves

Can't Beet it

- 2 carrots
- 2 kale leaves
- 1/2 beetroot
- 1/4 head of cabbage
- 1/4 bunch parsley
- 2 stalks celery
- 1 garlic clove (optional)

Carrots 4 Breakfast Juice

- 1" slice of ginger
- 4 carrots
- 1 apple (cored)
- 1 lemon

Carrot-Kale Combo

- 1 green apple (cored)
- 3 handfuls spinach
- 6 kale leaves
- 4 large carrots
- 1" slice of ginger

Daily Prayer Drink - Wren Archer

- 1 cup of plain Kefir with Omega 3 tropical fruit flavored clarified fish oil
- 1 teaspoon of raw Manuka Honey
- A splash of mineral water to loosen it up
-

Gazpacho Juice

- 4 plum tomatoes
- 1 large cucumber
- 2 stalks celery
- 1 red bell pepper
- 1/4 small red onion
- 2 cups parsley, leaves and stems
- 1 lime

Great Green Fruity Mix

- 2 cups beet greens
- 2 cups red Swiss chard
- 2 cups kale
- 2 cups spinach
- 1 apple (cored)
- 1/2 Comice pear
- 10 strawberries (green tops cut off)
- 1 cup coconut water

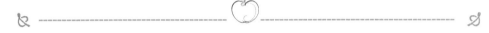

Great Greens Juice

- 2 green apples (cored)
- 2-3 cups spinach
- 6-8 leaves Swiss chard
- 1 cucumber
- 4 stalks celery
- 1/2 fennel bulb
- 1 bunch basil

Green Juice

- 6 leaves kale
- 2 cups spinach
- 1/2 cucumber
- 4 stalks celery
- 2 apples (cored)
- 1" slice of ginger root

Green Lemonade

- 1 green apple (cored)
- 3 handfuls spinach (approx. 1-1/2 cups)
- 6-8 kale leaves (approx. 2 cups)
- 1/2 cucumber
- 4 celery stalks
- 1/2 lemon

Green-Orange-Red Juice

- 1 cup spinach
- 3 celery stalks
- 1 red bell pepper
- 3 carrots
- 1 cucumber
- 1 garlic clove (optional)

Joe Ann's AM Cocktail – Serve over crushed ice. Makes 40 oz.

- ½ cup fresh black berries
- ½ cup fresh blueberries
- 1 dozen red grapes
- ½ cup dried plums
- 1 delicious apple (cored)
- 1 honey crisp apple
- 3 fresh pineapple wedges
- 1 frozen banana
- ½ c dried Craisins
- ½ tsp. Guarana powder
- 1 tbsp. hempseed
- 1 tsp. flaxseeds
- 1 tbsp. local honey
- 1 cup coconut milk

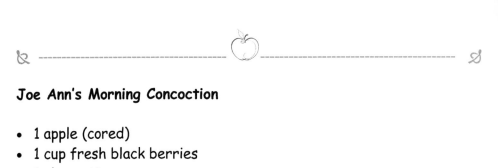

Joe Ann's Morning Concoction

- 1 apple (cored)
- 1 cup fresh black berries
- 1 clementine
- 3 fresh pineapple wedges
- handful of red grapes
- 1/2 cup almonds
- 1 banana
- 1/2 cup oatmeal
- 1 heaping Tbsp. coconut oil
- 1 Tbsp. flaxseed
- 1 cup ice cubes (made from coconut water)
- 1/2 cup coconut milk
- 1 tsp. Green Memory (can get this at health food stores)
- 1/2 tsp. Matcha powder (boosts immune system)

Juice Bunch

- 4 oz. tub alfalfa sprouts
- 4 carrots
- 3 stalks celery
- 1/2 bunch parsley
- 1/2 bunch spinach

Karen's Mean Green Juice

- 4-6 carrots
- 2 handfuls kale
- 5-6 celery stalks
- 1 radish bunch
- 1 green onion

Lean & Green Drink

- 1 tomato
- 4 carrots
- 2 green apples (cored)
- 1/2 bunch spinach
- 1/2 cucumber
- 1/2 lemon
- 2 celery stalks
- 6 kale leaves
- 2 sections grapefruit (peeled)
- 1 pear

Juice fruit together and place in blender with:
- 1 avocado
- 1 Tbsp. flax seed
- 1 Tbsp. hemp seed

Blend well.

Lemon Lime
- 1 lemon
- 1 lime
- 2 Asian pears
- 2 green apples (cored)
- 2 carrots
- 1" slice of ginger root
- 2 cups purple cabbage

Luscious Fruit Juice

- 2 oranges
- 2 green apples (cored)
- 1/4 grapefruit (I take the skin off and it's not as bitter)
- 1 sweet red apple (cored)

Juice fruit together and put in blender with:
- 6-8 frozen strawberries
- 1-2 frozen bananas (if I have it)
- 1 Tbsp. Hemp seeds
- 1 Tbsp. flax seeds
- 1 Tbsp. coconut oil

Mango Salsa Juice – Karen Clark

- 1 mango
- 1/2 cucumber
- 1/4 yellow pepper (capsicum)
- 1/2 jalapeno pepper
- 2 green onions or scallions (shallots)
- 1/4 cup cilantro (fresh coriander)
- 1/2 lime

*To make the juice less spicy remove ribs and seeds from Jalapeno pepper

Mexican-Style Juice

- 2 large cucumbers
- 4 cups cilantro, leaves and stems
- 1 lime
- 1 Poblano pepper, ribs and seeds removed
- 1 golden delicious apple (cored)

Minty-Fresh Berry

- 2 cups blueberries
- 2 kiwi fruit (peeled)
- 16 strawberries
- 2 cups mint leaves, packed into the measuring cup

Not Your Typical V8

- 4 tomatoes
- 3 carrots
- 1 green pepper
- 1/2 bunch spinach
- 4 green onions
- 1 lemon
- 2 celery stalks
- 1/2 bunch parsley

One Lonely Fruit

- 1/2 cucumber
- 2 stalks celery
- 2 large kale leaves
- 1/2 bunch spinach
- 1 kiwi

One-Two-Three-Four Juice

- 1 apple (cored)
- 2 beets
- 3 large carrots
- 4 cups spinach/kale
- 1" piece of ginger

Purple Power Juice

- 6 cups Concord grapes
- 1 Golden Delicious apple (cored)
- 1" piece of ginger
- 1/2 cup blackberries

Refreshing Fennel-Pear

- 2 Comice pears
- 2 medium fennel bulbs

Spinach-Fennel-Cucumber

- 1 fennel bulb
- 1 cucumber
- 3 celery stalks
- 3 cups spinach

Stomach Soother

- 1/2 head of cabbage (pulp can be used for coleslaw)
- 1 beetroot with the greens
- 2 large kiwis (peeled)

Sunset In A Glass

- 1 large sweet potato
- 1 medium carrot
- 1 red bell pepper
- 2 large red beets
- 2 Golden Delicious apples (cored)
- 1 orange

Sweet N Tart Citrus

- 3 cups cranberries
- 2 pieces of ginger (1")
- 3 oranges
- 2 small ruby red grapefruit
- 2 limes

Sweet Treat

* Because it's high in sugar, this one's best to use as a treat or for breakfast.

- 2 cups strawberries
- 2 cups blueberries
- 1 cup black cherries
- 3 carrots
- 1 tsp. cinnamon

Sweet Veggies

- 3 carrots
- 1/2 bunch spinach
- 1 cucumber
- 1/2 bunch broccoli
- 1/2 sweet potato
- 1 garlic clove (optional)

V28

- 3 large red beets
- 2 medium carrots
- 2 stalks celery
- 4 plum tomatoes
- 4 cups parsley, leaves and stems (roughly chopped and packed into the measuring cup)
- 1 jalapeno, ribs and seeds removed
- 12 red radishes

Substitutions

Mango: papaya, pineapple
Cucumber: zucchini (courgette), celery
Yellow pepper: red, green, orange pepper (capsicum), tomato
Jalapeno: any hot pepper (Serrano, habanero, Poblano, Anaheim, etc...)
Scallion (shallot): red or yellow onion, leeks, garlic
Cilantro (coriander): parsley

Almond milk

Almond milk is a great alternative to dairy milk and a healthy component for any smoothie or shake. Almonds are gluten-free, low in carbs, and promote a good cholesterol balance.

Ingredients:
- 1.5 cups raw almonds (unsalted, uncooked)
- 4 cups of filtered or spring water
- 1 vanilla bean, scoop out the seeds, or 1/2 teaspoon vanilla extract

Instructions:
- Soak the almonds in water at least 8 hours, up to about 12 hours; drain.
- Blend the almonds in 4 cups of fresh spring or filtered water; add the vanilla extract; blend until well mixed. If you want to sweeten the almond milk, honey, agave nectar or another reasonably healthy sweetener.
- Strain using a very fine strainer or sieve, a coffee filter, or several layers of cheesecloth (muslin); pour the almond milk through the filter into a large bowl underneath. Squeeze remaining pulp to remove liquid. The almond pulp left over can be dried and used to add more fiber to your diet (try it on your cereal or as a topping on a dessert.

  Almond milk can be kept in the refrigerator for 4-7 days, covered. Shake well before serving.

Coconut Milk Whipped Cream

Ingredients:
- One 15-ounce can full-fat coconut milk
- 1 tablespoon sugar or more to taste (*optional*)
- 1 teaspoon vanilla or more to taste (*optional*)

Instructions:

1. Place the can of coconut milk in the refrigerator and leave it there until well-chilled; overnight preferably.

2. Scoop out the firm waxy layer of cream that has solidified, leaving only the liquid. (You can use the water in smoothies, or just drink it straight.) Place the cream in a bowl and using a mixer whip the cream for 3-5 minutes until light and fluffy with soft peaks. Add sugar or vanilla, if using.

Herbs Aren't Just for Cooking!

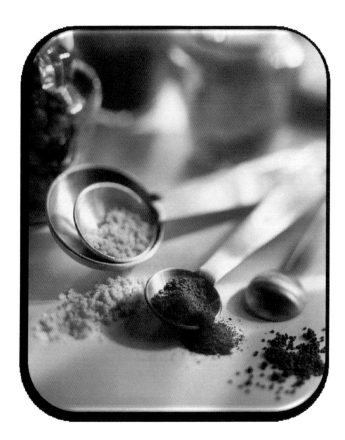

Add herbs and spices to your juice for extra nutrients
and flavor!

Basil

o Anti-inflammatory and anti-bacterial properties. Oil of basil herb has also been found to have anti-infective functions.

Black Cohosh

o For PMS and menopause symptoms like hot flashes and vaginal dryness, hormone levels, menstrual cramps, insomnia, arthritis, neuralgia, sciatica, cough and mucus reduction.

Borage

o For joint health, immunity, healthy skin and mucus membranes. Contains high levels of Vitamin A, Vitamin C, and iron. A good source of B-complex vitamins, and particularly rich in niacin (vitamin B-3).

Cayenne

o For circulatory system, cluster and migraine headaches, rheumatoid arthritis and bursitis, heartburn, cramps, and gas, obesity, psoriasis (topical), shingles and neuralgia, pain (topical).

Celery Seed

o For digestive aid, anxiety, detoxification, joint pain, rheumatism, arthritis, gout, blood pressure and cholesterol, urinary tract, menstrual discomforts, antiseptic and diuretic properties.

Chamomile

o For relaxation, insomnia, nerves, anxiety, menstrual cramps, irritable bowel syndrome (IBS), digestive ailments, diverticular disorders, canker sores, gingivitis, eczema.

Chia Seeds

o Truly a super seed! Adding just 2 tablespoons of chia seeds to your daily diet will give you approximately 7 grams of fiber, 4 grams of protein, 205 milligrams of calcium, and a whopping 5 grams of omega-3!

Cinnamon

o Can lower blood sugar, triglycerides, LDL, and total cholesterol in people with type 2 diabetes. Aim for one-fourth to one-half teaspoon of cinnamon twice a day. Good for diarrhea, ulcers, colic, indigestion, menstrual disorders, rheumatism, antifungal, antibacterial.

Coconut Oil

o For hair care, skin care, stress relief, maintaining cholesterol levels, weight loss, increased immunity, proper digestion and metabolism, relief from kidney problems, heart diseases, high blood pressure, diabetes, HIV and cancer, dental care, and bone strength. These benefits of coconut oil can be attributed to the presence of lauric acid, capric acid and caprylic acid, and its properties such as antimicrobial, antioxidant, antifungal, antibacterial, soothing, etc.

Coconut water

o High potassium content and contains antioxidants linked to a variety of health benefits such as aiding in digestion. Freeze coconut water in ice cube trays to add to your juice for extra health benefits.

Dandelion

o For detoxification, eczema, digestive system, liver, mild laxative, and an appetite stimulant.

Echinacea

o For colds, flu, and respiratory system, antiviral, anti-inflammatory, antibacterial, infection resistance.

Evening Primrose

o For breast pain (mastalgia), PMS, menopause ailments, arthritis, eczema, psoriasis, and acne, bruises, hemorrhoids, and an anti-inflammatory.

Feverfew

o For joints and rheumatoid arthritis, migraine headaches, aches and pains, anti-inflammatory, fever, menstrual cramps, and blood clot inhibition.

Flaxseed

o For nerve function, antibacterial, antifungal, antiviral properties, respiratory and cardiovascular systems, cholesterol and blood pressure, skin, hair, and nails, acne, eczema, psoriasis, and rosacea, high source of fiber, digestive aid, menstruation and hormonal balance.

Garlic

o Shown to destroys cancer cells and may disrupt the metabolism of tumor cells. Studies suggest that one or two cloves weekly provide cancer-protective benefits.

Ginger

o Can decrease motion sickness and nausea, may also relieve pain and swelling associated with arthritis. Ginger can also hinder blood clotting, so if you're about to have surgery or are taking blood thinners or aspirin, be sure to talk to your doctor first.

Ginseng

o For physical and mental vigor, for depression caused by exhaustion and stress, longevity and normalization of body functions, anti-inflammatory effects, mild stimulation, cholesterol and blood sugar, appetite and digestive stimulant, nausea, coughs, and respiratory system.

Grape Seed

o For antioxidant, diuretic, immune system, skin wounds, circulation, cholesterol collagen, skin tone, and elasticity, varicose veins, allergies, and macular degeneration, and arthritis.

Grapefruit

o For arterial health, cholesterol and triglycerides, antioxidant, digestive aid, weight loss, and psoriasis.

Green Tea

o For weight loss, detoxification, cholesterol, triglycerides, and blood pressure, appetite suppressant, tooth and gum health, immune system, energy, depression, and headaches.

Guarana

o For energy, mental alertness, fatigue; stamina and physical endurance, appetite suppressant, PMS headaches, astringent, and also a diuretic.

Hawthorn

o For cardiovascular system, hypertension, and has antioxidant properties.

Hemp Seeds

o One of the best sources of easily digestible plant protein above all nuts, seeds, and plants (aside from spirulina). Great for vegans who need protein!

Hops
- For digestive aid, insomnia, mild sedative effects, anxiety, skin injuries, muscle spasms and nerve pain.

Marshmallow
- For coughs, sore throats, skin inflammations, digestive tract, indigestion, GERD, diarrhea, inflammatory bowels, anti-inflammatory properties, and respiratory system.

Milk Thistle
- For detoxification, antidote to poisonous mushrooms, liver, spleen, gallstones, jaundice, antioxidant, and anti-inflammatory properties.

Nettle
- For allergies, hay fever, arthritis, hair growth stimulant, benign prostatic hyperplasia (BPH), coughs, and tuberculosis, and has anti-inflammatory properties.

Oregano
- A USDA study found that, gram for gram; oregano has the highest antioxidant activity of 27 fresh culinary herbs.

Paprika
- Contains capsaicin, which anti-inflammatory and antioxidant effects that may lower the risk of cancer No specific recommended dose, but moderation is probably the best way to go.

Peppermint
- For digestive aid, indigestion and colic, flatulence, and irritable bowel syndrome.

Psyllium
- For appetite suppressant, constipation, diarrhea, ulcerative colitis, irritable bowel syndrome (IBS), cholesterol, blood sugar, and blood pressure, hemorrhoids, and diverticulitis.

Rose Hips
- For antioxidant properties, urinary tract, bladder, headaches, dizziness, skin, and a source of iron

Rosemary
- Stops gene mutations that could lead to cancer and may help prevent damage to the blood vessels that raise heart attack risk.

Sarsaparilla

o For diuretic, detoxification, hormonal balance, rheumatism, arthritis, psoriasis, eczema, herpes, syphilis, antifungal, anti-inflammatory, and antibacterial.

Saw Palmetto

o For immune system, anti-inflammatory, aphrodisiac, sexual desire, benign prostatic hyperplasia (BPH), urinary tract and flow, reproductive system and sexual function.

Skullcap

o For antispasmodic effects, mild sedative, insomnia, nervous system, anxiety and nervous tension, and convulsions.

Slippery Elm

o For anti-inflammatory, antioxidant, sore throat, cough, diarrhea, inflammatory bowels, Crohn's disease, ulcerative colitis, GERD, gastritis, heartburn, skin inflammations, and hemorrhoids.

Spirulina

o For immune system, cardiovascular system, cholesterol, triglycerides, blood pressure, memory and cognitive function, and hay fever.

St John's Wort

o For depression and anxiety, seasonal affective disorder, antibacterial, PMS and menopause ailments, sciatica, nervous disorders, wounds, eczema, burns, and hemorrhoids.

Suma

o For immune system, cardiovascular and reproductive systems, cholesterol, circulation, PMS and menopause, anemia, fatigue and exhaustion, and anti-cancer properties.

Turmeric

o For rheumatism, arthritis, circulation, cholesterol, blood sugar, indigestion, ulcerative colitis, ulcers, antibacterial, antiviral, anti-inflammatory, antioxidant, vision, and skin diseases.

Valerian

o For mild sedative, anxiety and nervous disorders, insomnia, digestion, and nervous system.

White Willow

- o For fever, headaches, body aches and pains, arthritis, rheumatism, bursitis, neuralgia, menstrual cramps, digestive system, gastrointestinal conditions, and an anti-inflammatory.

Wild Yam

- o For antioxidant properties, menstrual cramps, nerve pain, indigestion, nausea, colic, morning sickness, coughs as an expectorant, blood sugar and cholesterol.

Yellow Dock

- ▪ For mild laxative, digestive system, constipation, liver, jaundice, psoriasis, eczema, hemorrhoids, and scurvy.

Additional Info:

- **Spirulina** is a type of blue-green algae that is rich in protein, vitamins, minerals, carotenoids, and antioxidants that can help protect cells from damage. It contains nutrients, including B complex vitamins, beta-carotene, vitamin E, manganese, zinc, copper, iron, selenium, and gamma linolenic acid (an essential fatty acid). Spirulina -- like any blue-green algae -- can be contaminated with toxic substances called microcystins. It can also absorb heavy metals from the water where it is grown. For these reasons, it is important to buy spirulina from a trusted brand.
- **Beetroot** – strong so only use ½ and your urine will be pink!
- **Cucumber juice** – helps rid the body of uric acid
- **Carrot juice** if you drink a lot everyday your skin will start to turn slightly orange!

Deficiency Signs & Symptoms

Tissue/ORGAN	SYMPTOM	POSSIBLE NUTRITIONAL DEFICIENCY OR TOXICITY
Mouth	Bleeding gums	Vitamin C deficiency
	Loose teeth	Advanced vitamin C deficiency (scurvy)
	Cracked lips + swollen, dark red tongue	Riboflavin (Vitamin B$_2$) deficiency
	Swollen dark red tongue	Biotin deficiency
	Sore tongue (glossitis)	Deficiencies in B12, folate, zinc or iron
	Pale tongue	Low iron levels
	Tooth decay	Deficiencies in B6, minerals (especially silica, calcium, boron)
	Bleeding gums	Deficiencies in vitamin C and bioflavonoids
	Cracks at the corners of the mouth	Deficiencies in B2 (riboflavin) or B-complex
Throat	Goiter	Iodine deficiency, autoimmune induced loss of thyroid function (hypothyroid)
Cardiovascular	Hypertension	Excess sodium, lack of calcium & potassium, excess body weight & poor physical conditioning, also genetic causes
	Atherosclerosis (blocked circulation)	High fat (especially saturated) diet often accompanied by obesity
	Poor circulation	Capillary damage due to poorly regulated diabetes
	Heart attack	See atherosclerosis
	Stroke	See hypertension, atherosclerosis
Respiratory	Asthma	A genetically increased requirement for vitamins E & C, may accompany food allergies
	Cancer	Possible deficiency of antioxidants & phytochemicals found in produce, exposure to environmental toxins, including those found in some foods, genetic component with some cancers, e.g. colon and ovarian

TISSUE/ORGAN	SYMPTOM	POSSIBLE NUTRITIONAL DEFICIENCY OR TOXICITY
Hair (on head)	Depigmentation of hair	Protein deficiency
	Flag sign: Stripes of de-pigmented hair	Transient, reoccurring protein deficiency
	Hair loss	Biotin deficiency, Folate, B5, B6, B-complex, and EFA deficiencies. Vitamin A toxicity or other environmental toxicity also causes hair loss.
	Dry, Brittle hair	Iodine deficiency, Essential fatty acid (EFA) deficiency
	Premature graying	Pantothenic acid (B5) deficiency.
	Dandruff	Deficiencies in EFA, antioxidants (selenium especially), B6 or B-complex. May also indicate low stomach acid.
Hair (body)	Profuse, long body hair (lanugo)	Anorexia
Eyes	Night blindness	Vitamin A or zinc deficiency
	Xerophthalmia (dry eyes)	Advanced vitamin A deficiency
	Macular degeneration	Age + lack of xanthene, an antioxidant from the carotene family commonly found in pumpkin, summer squash, and dark green vegetables.
	Retinal degeneration	Excess blood sugar (common in poorly regulated diabetes)
	Yellow "whites"	Jaundice from liver disease, excessive beta-carotene intake
	Dark circles under	Low levels of quercetin, vitamin C, and cromolyn for help with allergies. May indicate iron deficiency
	Floaters	Deficiencies in vitamin K, vitamin C, and bioflavonoids.
Ears	Excess ear wax	Low essential fatty acids (EFA)

TISSUE/ORGAN	SYMPTOM	POSSIBLE NUTRITIONAL DEFICIENCY OR TOXICITY
Liver	Failure	Alcohol toxicity, poisonous foods & herbs, e.g. some mushrooms, excess use of supplements such as vitamins A, D, B_6, and niacin
	Fatty	Early stages of alcoholism or genetics
	Gallstones	High fat diet + obesity, especially in overweight women of reproductive age
Kidneys	Damage	Exposure to environmental toxins, including those in some foods, excess nutrients such as fluoride
	Failure	Hyperglycemia due to poorly regulated diabetes, high protein diets
	Stones	Excess calcium
Pancreas	Pancreatitis	Alcoholism
	Autoimmune damage (insulin dependent diabetes)	Elevated blood glucose
	Cystic fibrosis	Nutrient deficiencies due to lack of digestive enzymes
Gastrointestinal tract	Constipation	Lack of dietary fiber, dehydration
	Colon cancer	Lack of dietary fiber, antioxidant deficiency, genetic predisposition
	Diarrhea	Deficiency of nutrients used to build intestinal lining, including protein, zinc, vitamin A, and B-complex vitamins
Urogenital tract	Recurrent bladder infections	May indicate lack of sufficient nutrients to build up a good lining
	Excess urination	Microbial infection, diabetes, excess caffeine consumption
	Insufficient urination	Dehydration Unusually colored urine Illness, excess intake of supplements such as vitamin C, riboflavin or carotenoid antioxidants
	Prostate cancer	Insufficient intake of the antioxidant lutein (the red pigment in tomatoes)
	Hypogonadism	Zinc deficiency in childhood

TISSUE/ORGAN	SYMPTOM	POSSIBLE NUTRITIONAL DEFICIENCY OR TOXICITY
Skeleton	Bowed legs, protruding breastbone (rickets)	Vitamin D deficiency during childhood
	Frequent fractures (osteomalacia)	Loss of calcium from bones due to adult vitamin D deficiency
	Pre-osteoporosis (osteopenia)	Weakened bones caused by lack of calcium during teen and adult years
	Osteoporosis	poor diet and age-related hormone changes
	Hypercalcification	Vitamin A toxicity
	Stunted growth	Starvation, protein deficiency
	Dwarfism	Possible zinc deficiency
Skin	Small red bumps on back of arms.	Deficiencies in vitamin A, vitamin E, zinc or EFA. Malabsorption of nutrients may be the cause
	Easy bruising	Deficiencies in vitamin K, C, E, or bioflavonoids
	Pellagra (dry, black skin)	Niacin (vitamin B_3) deficiency
	Dry, scaly skin	Essential fatty acid, vitamin E, or biotin deficiency
	Greasy, scaly skin	Riboflavin (B_2) deficiency
	Dry, stays peaked when pinched	Dehydration (water deficiency or electrolyte imbalance)
	Unusual skin rash	Excess supplement use, vitamin B_6 deficiency
	Skin tags around neck, arms and back	Glucose intolerance or reactive insulin levels. May be one of the first signs of blood sugar regulation problems.
Hands	Hang nails	Zinc deficiency.
	Skin cracking at tips	Deficiencies in zinc, vitamin E, or EFA.
	Cold hands	EFA, niacin (B3), vitamin E, B12 or iron. May be from anemia or Raynaud's syndrome.
Nails	Flat angle / spooning	Iron deficiency
	Cuticle inflammation	Zinc deficiency
	Ridging	Decreased minerals possibly from decreased stomach acid.
	Delayed wound healing	Vitamins C, A or zinc deficiency
	Calcification	Vitamin D toxicity
Neurological system	Numbness in extremities	Vitamin B_6 toxicity, vitamin B_1 deficiency (Beriberi)

Minerals

Mineral	Recommended Daily Allowance	Fruits	Vegetables	Nut/Grains
Calcium	Adults need 1000 mg/day. Children need 800 to 1300 mg/day.	Blackberries, Blackcurrants, Dates, Grapefruit, Mulberries, Oranges, Pomegranates, Prickly Pears	Amaranth leaves, Bok Choy, Brussels Sprouts, Butternut Squash, Celery, Chinese Broccoli, French Beans, Kale, Okra, Parsnip, Spirulina, Swiss Chard, Turnip	Almonds, Amaranth, Brazil Nuts, Filberts/Hazelnuts, Oats, Pistachios, Sesame Seeds, Wheat (Durum, Hard White)
Copper	The estimated safe and adequate intake for copper is 1.5 - 3.0 mg/day.	Avocado, Blackberries, Dates, Guava, Kiwi, Lychee, Mango, Passion fruit, Pomegranate	Amaranth leaves, Artichoke, French Beans, Kale, Lima Beans, Parsnip, Peas, Potatoes, Pumpkin, Spirulina, Winter Squash, Sweet Potato, Swiss Chard, Taro	Brazil Nuts, Buckwheat, Cashews, Chestnuts, Filberts/Hazelnuts, Oats, Sunflower Seeds, Walnuts, Wheat (Durum, Hard Red)
Iodine	Adults should get 150 mcgs per day. Children 70-150 mcg	Fruits grown in iodine-rich soils contain iodine.	Vegetables grown in iodine-rich soils contain iodine.	Nuts grown in iodine-rich soils contain iodine.

Mineral	Recommended Daily Allowance	Fruits	Vegetables	Nut/Grains
Iron .	Women and teenage girls (at least 15 mg a day) Men (can get by on 10) Children (10 to 12 mg) Vitamin C aids in absorption of iron. The tannin in non-herbal tea can hinder absorption of iron. Take iron supplements and your vitamin E at different times, the iron supplements will tend to neutralize the vitamin E. Vegetarians need to get twice as much dietary iron as meat eaters	Avocado, Blackberries, Blackcurrant, Boysenberries, Breadfruit, Cherries, Dates, Figs, Grapes, Kiwi, Lemon, Loganberries, Lychee, Mulberries, Passion Fruit, Persimmon, Pomegranate, Raspberries, Strawberry, Watermelon	Amaranth leaves, Bok Choy, Brussels Sprouts, Butternut Squash, French Beans, Kale, Leeks, Lima Beans, Peas, Potatoes, Pumpkin, Spirulina, Swiss Chard	Most nuts contain a small amount of iron. Amaranth, Buckwheat, Cashews, Coconut, Oats, Pine Nuts/Pignolias, Pumpkin Seeds, Rye, Spelt Wheat (Durum, Hard Red, Hard White)
Manganese	2.0-5.0 mg/day for adults 2.0-3.0 mg for children 7 - 10 1.5-2.0 mg for children 4 - 6 1.0-1.5 mg for children 1 - 3 0.6-1.0 mg for children 6 mos. - 1yr 0.3-0.6 mg for infants 0-6 months	Avocado, Banana, Blackberries, Blackcurrants, Blueberries, Boysenberries, Cranberries, Dates, Gooseberries, Grapefruit, Guava, Loganberries, Pineapple, Pomegranate, Raspberries, Strawberry	Amaranth leaves, Brussels Sprouts, Butternut squash French Beans, Kale, Leeks, Lima Beans, Okra, Parsnip, Peas, Potatoes, Spirulina, Winter Squash, Sweet Potato, Swiss Chard, Taro	Buckwheat, Coconut, Filberts/Hazel nuts, Macadamia Nuts, Oats, Pecans, Pine Nuts/Pignolias, Pumpkin, Seeds, Rice Brown, Rye, Spelt, Wheat (Durum, Hard Red, Hard White)

Mineral	Recommended Daily Allowance	Fruits	Vegetables	Nut/Grains
Magnesium	Adults need 310 to 420 mg/ day. Children need 130 to 240 mg/day.	Avocado, Banana, Blackberries, Blackcurrants, Breadfruit, Cherimoya, Dates, Guava, Kiwi, Loganberries, Mulberries, Passion Fruit, Pomegranate, Prickly Pear, Raspberries, Watermelon	Amaranth leaves, Artichoke, Butternut Squash, French Beans, Lima Beans, Okra, Peas, Spirulina, Swiss Chard	Almonds, Amaranth, Brazil Nuts, Buckwheat, Cashews, Oats, Peanuts, Pine Nuts/Pignolias, Pumpkin Seeds, Quinoa, Rye, Wheat (Durum, Hard Red, Hard White)
Phosphorous	Adults need 700 mg/day. Children need 500 to 1250 mg/day.	Avocado, Blackcurrants, Breadfruit, Dates, Guava, Kiwi, Lychee, Mulberries, Passion Fruit, Pomegranate	Amaranth leaves, Artichoke, Brussels Sprouts, Celeriac, Corn, French Beans, Lima Beans, Parsnip, Peas, Potatoes, Pumpkin, Spirulina, Taro	Brazil Nuts, Buckwheat, Cashews, Oats, Pine Nuts/Pignolias, Pumpkin Seeds, Quinoa, Rye, Spelt Sunflower Seeds, Wheat (Durum, Hard Red, Hard White)
Selenium	Men need 70 mcgs/day. Women need 55 mcgs/day.	Bananas, Breadfruit, Dates, Guava, Lychee, Mango, Passion Fruit, Pomegranate, Watermelon	Asparagus, Brussels Sprouts, French Beans, Lima Beans, Mushrooms, Parsnip, Peas, Spirulina	Amaranth, Barley, Brazil Nuts, Buckwheat, Cashews, Coconut, Rye, Wheat (Durum, Hard Red)
Sodium	500 mg/day for adults 120 mg for infants Daily Value recommendation - no more than 2,400 to 3,000 mg/day	Sodium occurs naturally in almost all fresh, whole fruits but passion fruit has a significant amount.	Amaranth leaves, Artichoke, Broccoli, Beetroot, Bok Choy, Brussels Sprouts, Celeriac, Celery, Fennel, Kale, Spirulina, Spaghetti Squash, Sweet Potatoes, Swiss Chard	Amaranth, Coconut, Pumpkin Seeds, Quinoa, Spelt

Vitamins

Vitamin	Recommended Daily Allowance	Fruits	Vegetables	Nut/Grains
A	10,000 IU/day (plant-derived) for adult males. 8,000 for adult females - 12,000 if lactating. 4,000 for children ages 1-3 5,000 for children ages 4-6 7,000 for children ages 7-10	Cantaloupes, Grapefruit, Guava, Mango, Papaya, Passion Fruit, Tomatoes, Watermelon	Amaranth Leaves, Bok Choy, Broccoli, Brussels Sprouts, Butternut Squash, Carrots, Chinese Broccoli, Chinese Cabbage, Kale, Leeks, Peas, Pumpkin, Rapini, Spinach, Summer and Winter Squash, Sweet Potato, Swiss Chard	Chestnuts, Pecans, Pistachios
B1 (Thiamine)	1.2 mg for adult males and 1.1 mg for women - 1.5 mg if lactating. Children need .6 to .9 mg of B1/thiamine per day.	Avocado, Boysenberries, Breadfruit, Cherimoya, Dates, Grapes, Grapefruit, Guava, Loganberries, Mango, Orange, Pineapple, Pomegranate, Watermelon	Asparagus, Brussels Sprouts, Butternut Squash, Corn, French Beans, Lima Beans, Okra, Parsnips, Peas, Potatoes, Spirulina, Sweet Potato	Brazil Nuts, Buckwheat, Cashews, Chestnuts, Flax Seed, Filberts/Hazelnuts, Macadamia Nuts, Millet, Oats, Peanuts, Pecans, Pine Nuts/Pignolias, Pistachios, Quinoa, Rice Brown, Rye, Spelt ,Wheat (Durum, Hard Red, Hard White)

Vitamin	Recommended Daily Allowance	Fruits	Vegetables	Nut/Grains
B6 (Pryidoxine)	1.3 to 1.7 mg for adults - 2 mg for women who are pregnant or lactating. Children need between 0.6 to 1.3 mg B6 per day.	Avocado, Banana, Breadfruit, Cherimoya, Dates, Gooseberries, Grapes, Guava, Lychee, Mango, Passion Fruit, Pineapple, Pomegranate, Watermelon	Amaranth Leaves, Bok Choy, Broccoli, Brussels Sprouts, Butternut Squash, Celeriac, Corn, French Beans, Green Pepper, Kale, Lima Beans, Okra, Peas, Potatoes, Spirulina, Spaghetti Squash, Winter Squash, Sweet Potato, Taro	Chestnuts, Filberts/Hazelnuts, Pistachios, Pumpkin Seeds, Rice Brown, Rye, Sunflower Seeds, Walnuts, Wheat (Durum, Hard Red, Hard White)
B9 (Folate/Folic Acid)	At least 400 mcgs for most adults - pregnant women 600 mcgs and breastfeeding women should get at least 500 mcgs. Children need between 150 to 300 mcg per day.	Avocado, Blackberries, Boysenberries, Breadfruit, Cherimoya, Dates, Guava, Loganberries, Lychee, Mango, Orange, Papaya, Passion Fruit, Pineapple, Pomegranate, Raspberries, Strawberries	Amaranth Leaves, Artichoke, Asparagus, Beetroot, Bok Choy, Broccoli, Brussels Sprouts, Chinese Broccoli, Chinese Cabbage, French Beans, Lima Beans, Okra, Parsnip, Peas, Potatoes, Spinach, Spirulina, Summer & Winter Squash	Buckwheat, Chestnuts, Filberts/Hazelnuts, Oats, Peanuts, Quinoa, Rye, Sunflower Seeds, Wheat (Durum, Hard Red, Hard White)

Vitamin	Recommended Daily Allowance	Fruits	Vegetables	Nut/Grains
C	60 mg for adults - 70 mg for women who are pregnant and 95 for those lactating. Children need between 45 and 50 mg	Black Currants, Breadfruit, Grapefruit, Guava, Kiwi, Lychee, Mango, Mulberries, Orange, Papaya, Passion Fruit, Pineapple, Strawberries	Amaranth Leaves, Bok Choy, Broccoli, Brussels Sprouts, Butternut Squash, Green Pepper, Kale, Swiss Chard	Other than Chestnuts, most nuts do not contain a significant amount of vitamin C.
E	30 IU for most adults. Children need between 6-11 mg/day. (1 IU is equal to approximately .75 mg)	Avocado, Blackberries, Black Currants, Blueberries, Boysenberries, Breadfruit, Cranberries, Guava, Kiwi, Loganberries, Mango, Mulberries, Nectarine, Papaya, Peach, Pomegranate, Raspberries	Butternut Squash, Parsnip, Potatoes, Pumpkin, Spirulina, Swiss Chard, Taro	Almonds, Filberts/Hazelnuts, Pine Nuts/Pignolias, Sunflower Seeds
K	70-80 micrograms/day for adult males, 60-65 micrograms per day for adult females. Children need about half the amount, depending on age.	Avocado, Blackberries, Blueberries, Boysenberries, Chinese Pear, Cranberries, Grapes, Kiwi, Loganberries, Mango, Mulberries, Pear, Plum, Pomegranate, Raspberries, Tomatoes	Alfalfa, sprouted, Artichoke, Asparagus, Bok Choy, Broccoli, Brussels Sprouts, Cabbage, Carrots, Cauliflower, Celery, Chinese Broccoli, Cucumber, Kale, Leeks, Okra, Peas, Rapini Spinach, Spirulina, Winter Squash , Swiss Chard	Cashews, Chestnuts, Filberts/Hazelnuts, Pine Nuts/Pignolias, Pistachios, Rye

Metric to US Conversions	MEASUREEQUIVALENT
1 milliliter	1/5 teaspoon
5 ml	1 teaspoon
15 ml	1 tablespoon
30 ml	1 fluid oz.
100 ml	3.4 fluid oz.
240 ml	1 cup
1 liter	34 fluid oz.
1 liter	4.2 cups
1 liter	2.1 pints
1 liter	1.06 quarts
1 liter	.26 gallon
1 gram	.035 ounce
100 grams	3.5 ounces
500 grams	1.10 pounds
1 kilogram	2.205 pounds
1 kilogram	35 oz.

US Dry Volume Measurements	MEASURE EQUIVALENT
1/16 teaspoon	dash
1/8 teaspoon	a pinch
3 teaspoons	1 Tablespoon
1/8 cup	2 tablespoons (1 standard coffee scoop)
1/4 cup	4 Tablespoons
1/3 cup	5 Tablespoons + 1 teaspoon
1/2 cup	8 Tablespoons
3/4 cup	12 Tablespoons
1 cup	16 Tablespoons
1 Pound	16 ounces

US liquid volume measurements	MEASURE EQUIVALENT
8 Fluid ounces	1 Cup
1 Pint	2 Cups (16 fluid ounces)
1 Quart	2 Pints (4 cups)
1 Gallon	4 Quarts (16 cups)

US to Metric Conversions	MEASUREEQUIVALENT
1/5 teaspoon	1 ml (ml stands for milliliter, one thousandth of a liter)
1 teaspoon	5 ml
1 tablespoon	15 ml
1 fluid oz.	30 ml
1/5 cup	50 ml
1 cup	240 ml
2 cups (1 pint)	470 ml
4 cups (1 quart)	.95 liter
4 quarts (1 gal.)	3.8 liters
1 oz.	28 grams
1 pound	454 grams

Sugar	Sugar Substitute
2 cups Sugar	1 cup of Honey
2 cups Sugar	1 cup of Molasses
1 cup Sugar	1/2 cup Maple Syrup
1 cup Sugar	1/4 cup Maple Sugar
1 cup Sugar	1/2 cup Agave Nectar
1 cup Sugar	1 cup Coconut Sugar
1 cup Sugar	1/8 cup Stevia
1 cup Sugar	1/4 + 1/8 cup Xylitol (6 Tbsp.)

Index

Don't put the responsibility of your health on anyone but yourself! I've found out so much about processed foods doing this book that I honestly can't eat a lot of things anymore.

The FDA has a pamphlet called "Defect Levels Handbook" regarding the amount of bugs, rat hairs and grit that are allowed in our foods! Don't believe me? You can find it here:

http://www.fda.gov/food/guidancecomplianceregulatoryinformation/guidancedocuments/sanitation/ucm056174.htm

Here's a good article on what's in juice purchased at stores:

http://www.foodrenegade.com/secret-ingredient-your-orange-juice/

Made in the USA
Lexington, KY
05 February 2013